Ken Grauer, M.D., F.A.A.F.P.
Professor,
Department of Community Health and Family Medicine;
Assistant Director,
Family Practice Residency Program,
University of Florida, College of Medicine,
Gainesville, Florida;
ACLS National Affiliate Faculty

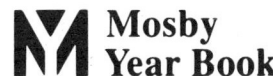

St. Louis   Baltimore   Boston   Chicago   London

Philadelphia   Sydney   Toronto

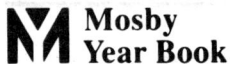
Mosby
Year Book

Dedicated to Publishing Excellence

Editor: Don Ladig
Developmental editor: Jeanne Rowland
Project manager: Mark Spann
Production editor: Stephen C. Hetager

Illustrations: Mark Swindle,
George Wassilchenko
Cover art: © George Wassilchenko

Copyright © 1992 by Mosby–Year Book, Inc.

All rights reserved. No part of this publication may be reproduced, stored in a retrieval system, or transmitted, in any form or by any means, electronic, mechanical, photocopying, recording, or otherwise, without prior written permission from the publisher.

Printed in the United States of America

Mosby–Year Book, Inc.
11830 Westline Industrial Drive
St. Louis, Missouri 63146

Library of Congress Cataloging in Publication Data

Grauer, Ken.
  ECG interpretation pocket reference / Ken Grauer.
    p. cm.
  Companion v. to: A practical guide to ECG interpretation/Ken Grauer. c1991.
    ISBN 0-8016-2002-3
  1. Electrocardiography—Interpretation—Handbooks, manuals, etc.
I. Grauer, Ken. Practical guide to ECG interpretation. II. Title
  (DNLM: 1. Electrocardiography—handbooks. WG 39 G774e)
RC683.5.E5G663 1991
616.1′207547—dc20
DNLM/DLC
for Library of Congress
91-27611
CIP

CL/PC 9 8 7 6

Preface

Electrocardiography is not difficult. At least it is *not* difficult to obtain a basic understanding of the art, and to be able to apply this understanding to the interpretation of the majority of 12-lead ECGs that you will encounter.

The most difficult part of electrocardiography is learning (and then remembering) the various criteria used to diagnose findings such as left ventricular hypertrophy and bundle branch block. Practically speaking, however, there is really much *less* to learn (and memorize) than most people think. *The secret lies with understanding and applying!* Herein lies the purpose of this pocket reference. After all,

> "Why memorize, when there are plenty of smart books around?"
>
> Lou Kuritzky

To emphasize this point, we have consolidated the basic core content of electrocardiography into this pocket reference. Selected tables and figures have been reproduced from our book *A Practical Guide to ECG Interpretation* (Grauer, K., Mosby-Year Book, 1992), and organized according to basic content areas, including a systematic approach to interpretation; determination of rate and rhythm; determination of intervals, axis, and bundle branch blocks and hemiblocks; chamber enlargement; and QRST changes. Pearls regarding more advanced concepts have also been included, such as criteria for diagnosis of infarction and ischemia, the five "Essential Lists," electrolyte disturbances, diagnosis of pericarditis, and pediatric norms.

We suggest you first familiarize yourself with the content of this pocket reference. After doing so, we encourage you to carry it with you in your daily practice, and refer to it whenever you encounter an ECG about which you have a question. Doing so should not only eliminate the need to memorize cumbersome tables and criteria, but also facilitate and improve your ECG interpretation ability, while at the same time making the process much more enjoyable.

Ken Grauer

Contents

The Systematic Approach, 1
Figure 2-1: *Mnemonic for systematic approach to ECG interpretation,* **1**
Helpful hints for applying the Systematic Approach, **1**

Rate & Rhythm, 5
Table 3-1: *The Four Key Questions of rhythm analysis,* **5**
Figures 3-2 and 3-3: *Calculation of heart rate,* **5**

A List of Common Arrhythmias, 7

The PR Interval, 11
Table 4-1: *Assessing the PR interval,* **11**

The QRS Interval/Bundle Branch Block, 12
Table 5-1: *Assessing QRS duration,* **12**
Figure 5-1: *Algorithm for assessment of QRS widening,* **13**
Figure 5-9: *Typical secondary ST-T wave changes of RBBB and LBBB,* **15**
Diagnosis of infarction in the presence of bundle branch block, **15**
Figure 5-8: *Diagnosis of typical RBBB, typical LBBB, and IVCD,* **14**
Figure 5-13: *Examples of variations of QRS morphology in lead V_1 in RBBB,* **14**

WPW, 16
Figure 5-14: *The characteristic findings in WPW,* **16**

The QT Interval, 17
Table 6-1: *Assessing the QT interval,* **17**
Figure 6-2: *Determining QT prolongation,* **18**

Axis (and Hemiblocks), 19
Table 7-1: *Rapid determination of axis deviation,* **20**
Figure 7-14: *The hexaxial lead system,* **19**
Table 7-2: *Determination of pathologic LAD,* **21**

Chamber Enlargement, 22
Table 9-1: *Simplified criteria for the ECG diagnosis of LVH,* **22**
Table 9-2: *Additional voltage criteria for the ECG diagnosis of LVH,* **22**
Figure 9-4: *Normal ST segment and T wave; "strain"; "strain equivalent pattern,"* **23**
Figure 9-2: *ECG criteria for diagnosis of RAA and LAA,* **24**
Table 9-3: *Findings suggestive of RVH in adults,* **25**
Table 9-4: *Findings suggestive of pulmonary disease in adults,* **25**

QRST Changes, 26
Table 10-1: *Suggested approach to systematically assessing QRST changes,* **26**
Table 10-2: *Basic lead groups,* **27**
Table 10-3: *Leads that may normally display moderate- to large-sized Q waves,* **27**
Table 10-6: *Leads that may normally display T wave inversion,* **28**

Figure 10-15: *"Smiley" vs "frowny" ST segment elevation,* **28**
Figure 10-16: *Examples of alterations in T wave morphology,* **29**
Figure 10-3: *Schematic view of the heart (showing normal R wave progression),* **30**
Table 10-4: *Common causes of poor R wave progression,* **31**
Figure 10-14: *Examples of ST segment elevation,* **31**

Infarction and Ischemia, 32

Table 12-1: *Information sought from the ECG in patients with chest pain,* **32**
Table 12-2: *General descriptors for dating infarction,* **33**
Figure 12-1: *Principal ECG indicators of acute infarction,* **34**
Figure 12-3: *Simplified diagram of the coronary circulation,* **35**
Table 12-3: *Criteria for considering thrombolytic therapy,* **35**
Table 12-4: *Patients likely to benefit most from thrombolytic therapy,* **36**

The Five Essential Lists, 37

Table 13-2: *List #1: Causes of a regular, wide-complex tachycardia,* **37**
Table 13-3: *List #2: Common causes of QT prolongation,* **38**
Table 13-4: *List #3: Common causes of ST segment depression,* **39**
Table 13-5: *List #4: Common causes of a tall R wave in lead V_1,* **39**
Table 13-6 *Helpful clues for determining the cause of a tall R wave in lead V_1,* **40**
Table 13-7: *List #5: Causes of anterior ST segment depression in the setting of acute inferior infarction.* **41**
Figure 13-12: *Application of the mirror test,* **42**

Electrolyte Disturbances, 44
Figure 14-1: *ECG manifestations of hyperkalemia,* **44**
Table 14-1: *Common clinical settings likely to produce hyperkalemia,* **44**
Figure 14-2: *ECG manifestations of hypokalemia,* **45**

Pericarditis, 46
Figure 15-1: *Stage 1 of acute pericarditis,* **46**
Figure 15-2: *Stage 3 of acute pericarditis,* **47**

Recognizing Lead Misplacement, 48
Table 16-1: *Findings suggestive of limb lead misplacement,* **48**
Figure 16-1: *Schematic illustration of lead misplacement in the standard leads,* **49**

When the Patient is a Child, 50
Table 17-2: *Normal rhythm and axis findings in children,* **50**
Table 17-1: *Pediatric norms for heart rate and intervals,* **51**
Table 17-3: *Greatly simplified voltage criteria for diagnosing RVH and LVH in children,* **52**

When 12 Leads are Better than One, 53
Table 19-1: *Reasons why 12 leads are better than one,* **54**
Figure 19B-4: *Differentiation of wide beats when the QRS complex is upright in V_1,* **56**
Figure 19B-5: *Differentiation of wide beats when the QRS complex is negative in V_1,* **56**

The Systematic Approach

The key to 12-lead ECG interpretation is to have a systematic approach (Figure 2-1):

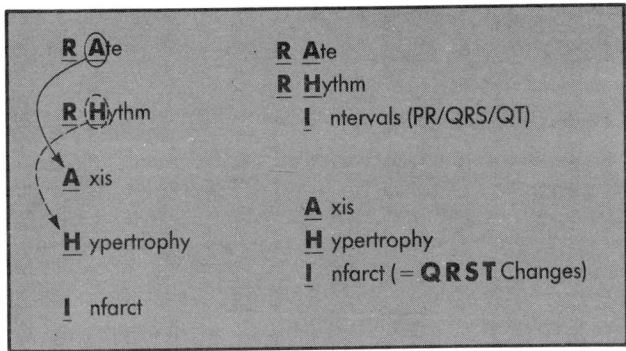

Figure 2-1. Mnemonic for systematic approach to ECG interpretation.

Helpful hints for applying the systematic approach:

RAte—Divide 300 by the number of boxes in the R-R interval. *(See Figures 3-2 and 3-3 on pp 5-6 in pocket reference.)*

Rhythm—Are there P waves? Are P waves "married" to the QRS? *(See Table 3-1 on p 5 in pocket reference.)*
   The P wave should always be upright in lead II if there is sinus rhythm—unless there is lead reversal or dextrocardia. (See pp 48-49 in pocket reference.)

Intervals—*Don't forget to look at intervals early in the process!* For practical purposes:
   The **PR interval** is normal if it *does not* exceed a large box. *(See Table 4-1 on p 11 in pocket reference.)*
   The **QRS Interval** should not be greater than *half* a large box. *(See Table 5-1 on p 12 in pocket reference.)*

If the QRS is wide, STOP and find out why (i.e., RBBB, LBBB, IVCD, or WPW) before proceding further! (See pp. ●●●-●●● in pocket reference.)

   The **QT interval** should be *less than half* the R-R interval (if the heart rate is under 100 beats/minute). *(See Table 6-1 and Figure 6-2 on pp 17-18 in pocket reference.)*

Axis—Concentrate on leads I and aVF (and perhaps II). For practical purposes:
   The axis is **normal** if net QRS deflection is positive in leads I and aVF.
   There is **RAD** if net QRS deflection is negative in lead I, but positive in lead aVF.
   There is **LAD** if net QRS deflection is positive in lead I, but negative in lead aVF *(and pathologic LAD = **LAHB** if net QRS deflection is negative in lead II)*.
   The axis is **indeterminate** if net QRS deflection is negative in leads I and aVF
   (See pp 19-21 in pocket reference.)

Hypertrophy—Look for signs of enlargement of the four chambers. For practical purposes:

The "magic numbers" for *LVH* are 35 (*deepest S in V_1 or V_2 PLUS tallest R in V_5 or V_6 in a patient $\geq$35 years of age*) **and 12** (*for the R in lead aVL*). LVH is much more likely to be present if in addition to voltage criteria, there is also **"strain"**!

There is *RAA* (*P-pulmonale*) if P waves are **p**rominent ($\geq$2.5 mm tall) and **p**eaked (i.e., *uncomfortable to sit on*) in the **p**ulmonary leads (II, III, and aVF).

There is *LAA* (*P-mitrale*) if P waves are notched (***M**-shaped*) in the **m**itral leads (I, II, or aVL), or if there is a deep terminal negative component to the P in lead V_1.

Consider ***pulmonary disease*** if there is RAA, RAD, or indeterminate axis, incomplete RBBB (or an rSr' pattern in lead V_1), low voltage, or persistent precordial S waves—and ***RVH*** if there is also a tall R wave in lead V_1 and right ventricular strain.

(*See pp 22-25 in pocket reference.*)

Infarct (= **QRST** changes)—*Look at all leads (except aVR) for:*

Q waves: Small (*normal septal q waves*) are commonly seen in lateral leads (I, aVL, V_4, V_5, and/or V_6); moderate- or large-sized Q waves may be normal (as an *isolated* finding) in leads III, aVF, aVL, and V_1.

R wave progression: Transition should occur between V_2 and V_4:
  Tall R wave in lead V_1? rSr' pattern in lead V_1?

ST segments: Concentrate more on shape (i.e., *"smiley"* or *"frowny"*) than on the *amount* of ST segment deviation,

T waves: May normally be inverted in leads III, aVF, aVL, and V_1.

(*See pp 26-31 in pocket reference.*)

*Use the above outline as a guide for your **descriptive analysis**; then formulate your **clinical impression**. Whenever possible, WRITE OUT your findings. (BUT even when time is short, ALWAYS be SYSTEMATIC in your approach!!!)*

Finally, remember the **Five Essential Lists** *(see pp 37-43 in pocket reference):*

List #1: Causes of a regular, wide-complex tachycardia (Table 13-2)

List #2: Common causes of QT prolongation (Table 13-3)

List #3: Common causes of ST segment depression (Table 13-4)

List #4: Common causes of a tall R wave in lead V_1 (Table 13-5)

List #5: Causes of anterior ST segment depression in the setting of acute inferior infarction (Table 13-7)

Rate & Rhythm

Table 3-1

The Four Key Questions of Rhythm Analysis

1. Is the rhythm regular?
2. Are there P waves?
3. Is the QRS wide or narrow?
4. "Who's married to whom?" (i.e., *Is the P related to the QRS?*)

Calculation of Heart Rate

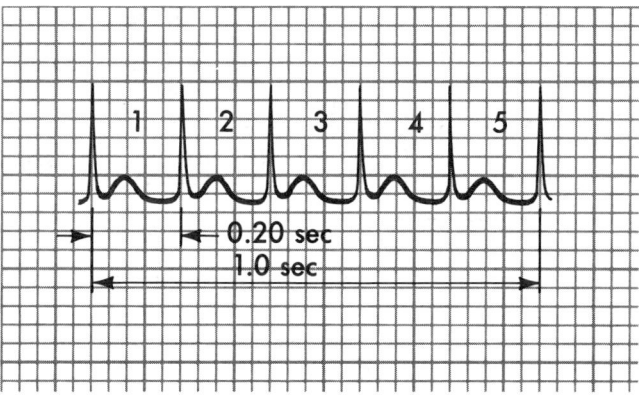

Figure 3-2. A QRS complex occurs each large box. The R-R interval is therefore 0.20 second, and the heart rate is 300 beats/minute.

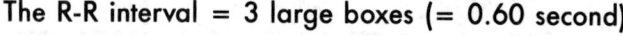
> If the rhythm is regular, heart rate can be estimated by dividing 300 by the number of large boxes in the R-R interval (Figure 3-3).

The R-R interval = 3 large boxes (= 0.60 second)

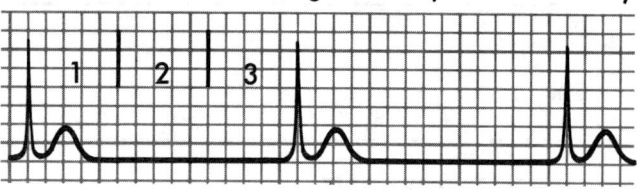

HR = 300 ÷ 3 = 100 beats/minute

The R-R interval = 4 large boxes (= 0.80 second)

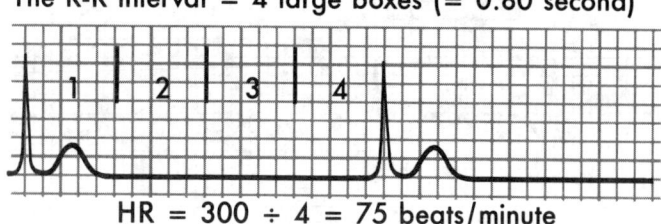

HR = 300 ÷ 4 = 75 beats/minute

Figure 3-3

A List of Common Arrhythmias

Sinus Mechanism Rhythms/Arrhythmias ($\Rightarrow$ *the P Wave is Upright in Lead II*)

Normal Sinus Rhythm (NSR): regular rhythm; rate between 60 and 99 beats/minute*

Sinus Bradycardia: regular rhythm; rate below 60 beats/minute*

Sinus Tachycardia: regular rhythm; rate 100 beats/minute or faster*

Sinus Arrhythmia: sinus mechanism; irregular rhythm

Other Supraventricular ($\Rightarrow$ *Narrow QRS*) Arrhythmias

Atrial Fibrillation: irregularly irregular rhythm; no definite P waves. By definition, it is impossible to specify the rate of atrial fibrillation (since the rate of this irregularly irregular rhythm changes from beat to beat). We feel it best to describe atrial fibrillation as having one of the following:

A rapid ventricular response—if the rate averages over 120 beats/minute

A controlled (moderate) ventricular response—if the rate averages between 70 and 110 beats/minute

A slow ventricular response—if the rate averages less than 60 beats/minute

---

*These norms are different for children *(see Table 17-1 on p 51 in pocket reference)*.

Atrial Flutter: regular atrial rate that is most often close to 300 beats/minute; characteristic *sawtooth* pattern (especially in the inferior leads). Most commonly there is a 2:1 ventricular response (atrial rate about 300 beats/minute ⇒ ventricular rate about 150 beats/minute); less commonly there is a 4:1 ventricular response (ventricular rate about 75 beats/minute)—though other ratios or an irregular ventricular response may also be seen.

PSVT (Paroxysmal SupraVentricular Tachycardia): regular supraventricular tachycardia at a rate of 150 to 240 beats/minute without obvious atrial activity (although sometimes subtle notching or a negative deflection representing retrograde atrial activity may be seen at the tail end of the QRS complex).

Formerly this rhythm was known as PAT or PJT (paroxysmal atrial or junctional tachycardia), but this older terminology implies more than we really know about the mechanism of the arrhythmia. In most cases in adults, PSVT is a **reentry** tachycardia that involves the AV node.

Junctional (AV Nodal) Rhythms: regular supraventricular rhythms in which the P wave in lead II is *negative* (preceding or following the QRS) or absent (see Figure 3-14 in *Practical Guide*).

AV Nodal Escape Rhythm—when the junctional rate is between 40 and 60 beats/minute and the rhythm arises because the SA node is delayed or fails in its pacemaking function

Accelerated Junctional Rhythm—when the junctional rate speeds up to between 61 and 99 beats/minute and takes over the pacemaking function

Junctional Tachycardia—when the junctional rate speeds up to over 100 beats/minute and takes over the pacemaking function

Premature Beats

Premature beats are beats that interrupt the underlying rhythm by occurring *earlier than expected*. They are of three types:

PACs (premature *atrial* contractions)—when the underlying rhythm is interrupted by an early beat arising from somewhere in the atria other than the SA node. Most often the impulse is conducted with a narrow QRS complex that is identical in appearance to that of normal sinus-conducted beats.

PJCs (premature *junctional* contractions)—when the underlying rhythm is interrupted by an early beat arising from the AV node. Most often the impulse is conducted with a narrow QRS complex that is *similar or identical* in appearance to that of normal sinus-conducted beats.

PVCs (premature *ventricular* contractions)—when the underlying rhythm is interrupted by an early beat arising from the ventricles. PVCs are wide and have an appearance quite different from that of normal sinus-conducted beats.

Ventricular (⇒ *Wide QRS*) Arrhythmias

Ventricular rhythms are usually regular (or fairly regular) rhythms that arise from a focus in the ventricles. As a result, the QRS complex is wide and very different in appearance from normal sinus-conducted beats. Ventricular rhythms may arise as *escape* rhythms (if supraventricular pacemakers fail), or as *usurping* rhythms (when they override the preexisting supraventricular rhythm). Atrial activity is absent, unrelated to the QRS complex, or retrograde.

Idioventricular Escape Rhythm—when the ventricular rate is between 30 and 40 beats/minute

AIVR (Accelerated IdioVentricular Rhythm)—when the ventricular rate is over 50 beats/minute, but less than 110 to 120 beats/minute. This is usually an escape rhythm.

Ventricular Tachycardia—when the ventricular rate is over 120 to 130 beats/minute. This is always a usurping rhythm.

Ventricular Fibrillation—a totally disorganized, chaotic ventricular rhythm. There is no meaningful perfusion with ventricular fibrillation.

The PR Interval

Table 4-1

Assessing the PR Interval

1. Verify that the patient is in sinus rhythm (by verifying that the P wave is upright in lead II). Measurement of the PR interval means little in the absence of a sinus mechanism.

2. If there is a sinus mechanism and the PR interval in lead II is:
   <0.12 second ⇒ The PR is short
   0.12 to 0.21 second ⇒ The PR is normal
   ≥0.22 second ⇒ The PR is long (= 1° AV block)

   > *Thus, the* **PR interval** *is* **short** *if it is less than three little boxes and* **long** *if it is clearly more than a large box!*

3. Precise measurement of a PR interval that falls within the normal range is not necessary. Clinically it suffices to say that the PR interval is "normal."

4. The limits given above do not necessarily hold true for children (for whom lesser degrees of PR prolongation are abnormal.

The QRS Interval/Bundle Branch Block

Table 5-1

Assessing QRS Duration

1. QRS duration can be measured from any of the 12 leads of a standard ECG.
2. All that matters is whether the QRS is normal or wide. Precise measurement of a QRS complex that is clearly of normal duration is unnecessary.
3. Judge QRS prolongation from the lead where the QRS appears to be longest.
4. If the QRS is:
    ≤0.10 second ⇒ The QRS is normal
    >0.10 second (i.e., clearly *GREATER* than half a large box) ⇒ The QRS is wide
5. The limits given above do not hold true for children (for whom lesser degrees of QRS prolongation are abnormal).

If the QRS is wide

If the QRS complex is wide, we suggest you *short-circuit* your systematic approach and immediately branch to the algorithm shown in Figure 5-1.

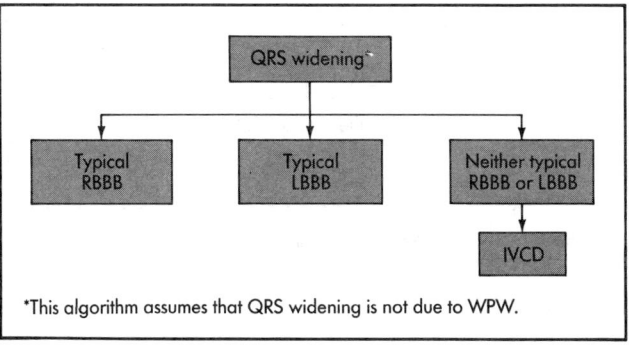

Figure 5-1. Algorithm for assessment of QRS widening.

Thus, if the QRS is wide, determine why *before* going any further.

Diagnosis of bundle branch block can be made from examination of the three *KEY* leads. The three KEY leads are I, V_1 and V_6. Practically speaking, these are the *ONLY* three leads you need to look at to diagnose RBBB and LBBB!

	Lead V$_1$	Leads I and V$_6$	QRS duration
Typical RBBB			≥0.11 sec
Typical LBBB			≥0.12 sec
IVCD	Neither typical RBBB nor LBBB morphology in the three key leads		≥0.11 sec

Figure 5-8. Diagnosis of typical RBBB, typical LBBB, and IVCD.

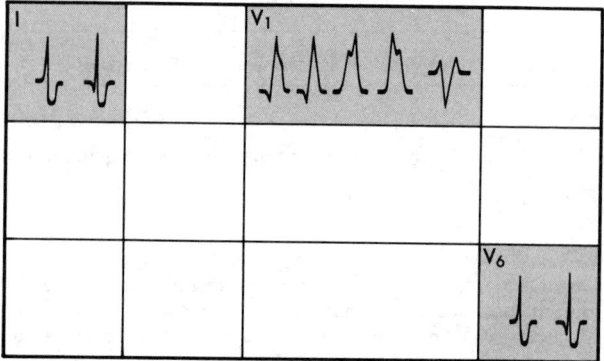

Figure 5-13. Examples of variations of QRS morphology in lead V$_1$ in RBBB.

Orientation of the ST segment and T wave with typical RBBB and LBBB is opposite that of the last QRS deflection in each of the three KEY leads.

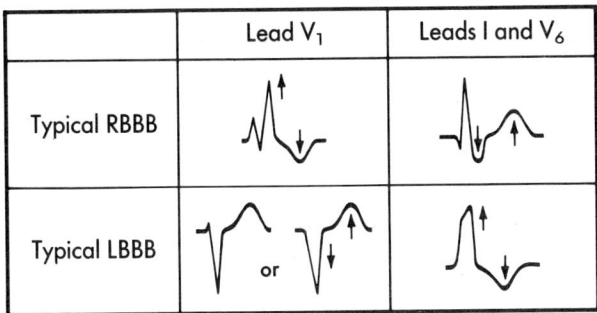

Figure 5-9. Typical secondary ST-T wave changes of RBBB and LBBB. The ST segment and T wave are oriented *opposite* to the direction of the last QRS deflection in these conduction defects.

Diagnosis of Infarction in the Presence of Bundle Branch Block

It is usually much harder to diagnose old or acute infarction in the presence of conduction abnormalities. Suspect infarction if you see:

A Q wave in leads I or V_6 in a patient with LBBB
Deep or wide Q waves in any leads with RBBB
Primary ST-T wave changes with bundle branch block
A *new* conduction defect in a patient with chest pain

WPW

There are three characteristic findings in WPW:

1. QRS widening
2. A delta wave
3. A short PR interval

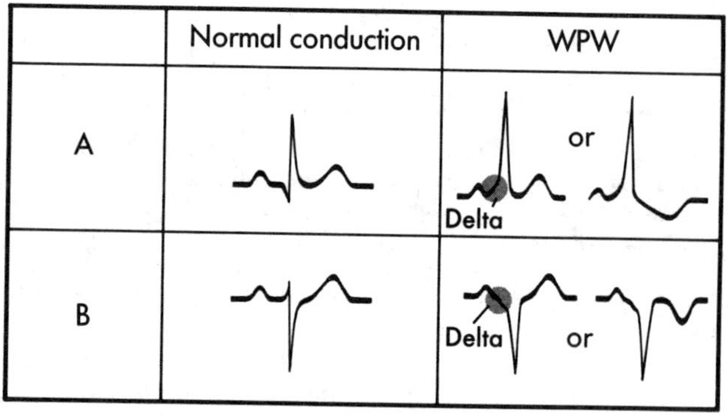

	Normal conduction	WPW
A		
B		

Figure 5-14. The characteristic findings in WPW (short PR interval, QRS widening, and delta wave), compared with normal conduction. **A** shows the usual appearance of WPW in leads where the QRS complex is predominantly upright, while **B** shows the appearance when the QRS complex is predominantly negative.

The QT Interval

Table 6-1

Assessing the QT Interval

1. Measure the QT interval from the onset of the Q wave (or the onset of the R wave if there is no Q) until the termination of the T wave.
2. Select a lead where you can clearly see the T wave.
3. Select the lead in which the QT interval appears to be longest.
4. Precise measurement of the QT interval is not necessary. Practically speaking, one only cares if the QT is normal or prolonged. In general, when the heart rate is under 100 beats/minute:

    If the QT is less than half the R-R interval ⇒ The QT is normal

    If the QT is clearly more than half the R-R interval ⇒ The QT is prolonged

    If the QT is about half the R-R interval ⇒ The QT is "borderline"

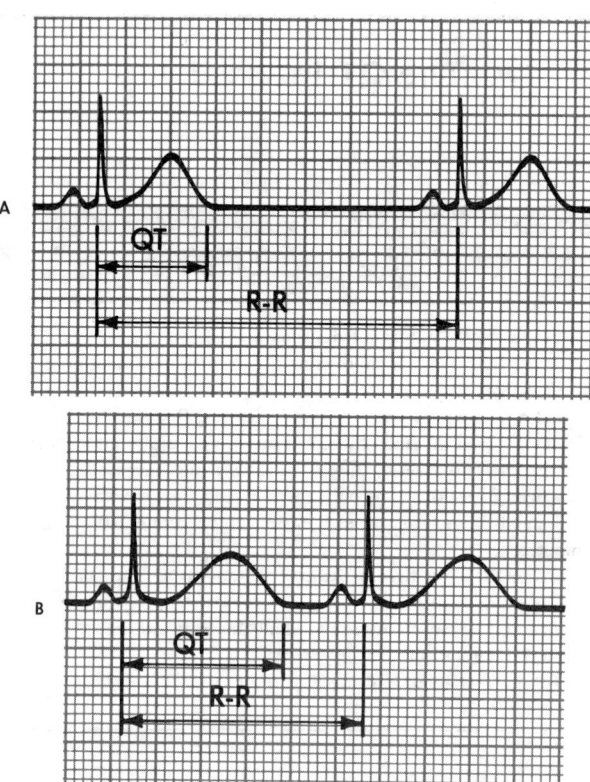

Figure 6-2. Determining QT prolongation. **A,** The QT interval is clearly normal, since the QT is much less than half the R-R interval. **B,** The QT is obviously prolonged. It far exceeds half the R-R interval.

Axis (and Hemiblocks)

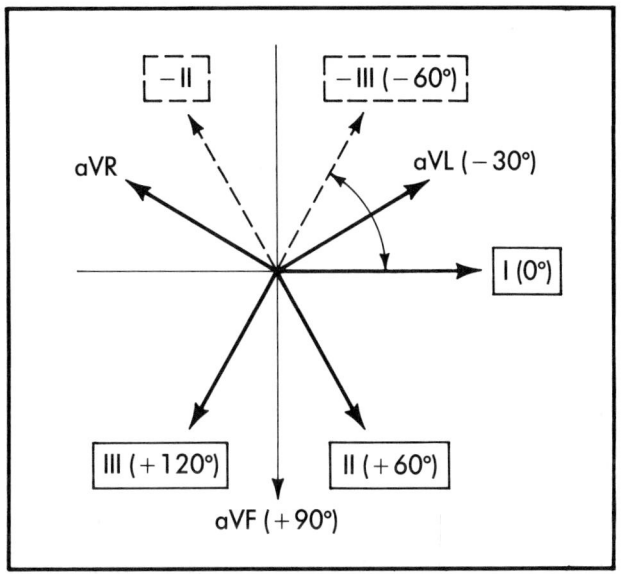

Figure 7-14. The hexaxial lead system. The **standard limb leads** (I, II, and III) are separated by 60°.

The three **augmented leads** are aVR, aVL, and aVF. Lead aVF is at +90°. Lead aVL bisects leads I and −III, and is at −30°. Lead aVR lies in "no-man's land." *Neither lead aVR nor lead aVL is essential to estimation of axis.*

Table 7-1

Rapid Determination of Axis Deviation

	Net QRS deflection	
	Lead I	**Lead aVF**
Normal axis	Positive	Positive
RAD	Negative	Positive
LAD	Positive	Negative
Indeterminate axis	Negative	Negative

Keep in mind that:

Lead I lies at 0° and lead aVF lies at 90°.

If the approximate size (i.e., net deflection) of lead I is about the same as that for lead aVF, then one would expect the axis to lie about midway between these leads (or close to +45°). We often give a range for our answer (i.e., *"The axis lies between +40° and +50°"*).

If the net deflection of lead I looks a lot greater than that for lead aVF, then the axis should lie closer to lead I (i.e., between 0° and +40°, depending on how much larger the net deflection in lead I looks to be).

If the net deflection of lead aVF looks a lot greater than that for lead I, then the axis should lie closer to lead aVF (i.e., between +50° and +90°, depending on how much larger the net deflection in lead aVF looks to be).

LAHB is far more common than LPHB. This is because the left posterior hemifascicle is much thicker than the anterior hemifascicle. It also has a dual blood supply (from the left and right coronary arteries), whereas the anterior hemifascicle does not.

For practical purposes, we equate the ECG diagnosis of LAHB with the finding of pathologic LAD. Thus, one only needs to look at lead II to make this diagnosis. *If the net deflection of lead II is negative, the axis is more negative than −30° and LAHB is present.*

Table 7-2

Determination of Pathologic LAD

1. If the net deflection in lead I is positive and lead aVF is negative, there is LAD (See Table 7-1).
2. To determine if this is pathologic LAD, look at QRS morphology in lead II:

Lead II	Axis	Pathologic LAD?
	Less negative than −30°	No
	−30°	Borderline
	More negative than −30°	Yes

Chamber Enlargement

Table 9-1

Simplified Criteria for the ECG Diagnosis of LVH

1. Deepest S wave in lead V_1 or V_2, *plus* tallest R wave in lead V_5 *or* V_6 ≥35
2. R in lead aVL ≥12
3. Patient ≥35 years old
4. "Strain"

Table 9-2

Additional Voltage Criteria for the ECG Diagnosis of LVH

1. An R wave ≥20 in any of the inferior leads (II, III, or aVF)
2. Deep S waves (≥20-25) in leads V_1 or V_2
3. An R wave ≥25 in lead V_5
4. An R wave ≥20 in lead V_6

What if There is a Conduction Defect?

Suspect LVH despite RBBB if the R wave in aVL ≥12, or R in V_5 or V_6 is ≥25.

Suspect LVH despite LBBB or IVCD if the S wave in V_1, V_2, or V_3 is ≥30.

Practically speaking, it is probably best not to even bother trying to diagnose RVH with LBBB, RBBB, or IVCD.

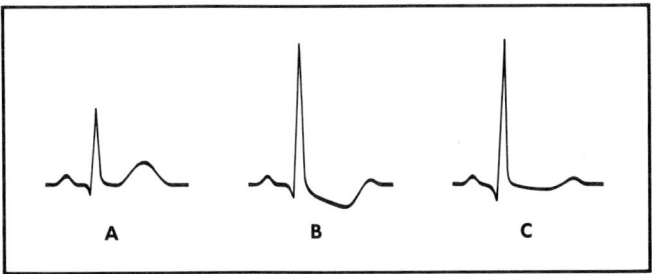

Figure 9-4. A, Normal ST segment and T wave. **B,** Asymmetric ST segment depression and T wave inversion characteristic of "strain." **C,** "Strain equivalent" pattern. Flattening of the T wave and/or slight ST segment depression with decreased T wave amplitude.

The leads most likely to demonstrate strain are the leads that look at the left ventricle (i.e., leads I, aVL, V_5, and V_6).

Condition	P Wave Appearance		Mnemonic Features
	Lead II	Lead V_1	
Normal Sinus Rhythm (NSR)	∧	∧ or ∨ or ∿	The P should be upright in lead II if there is sinus rhythm. The P wave may be upright, negative, or biphasic in lead V_1 with sinus rhythm
RAA (= **P P**ulmonale)	∧ 2.50		**P**rominent (≥ 2.5 mm tall) **p**eaked P waves in the **p**ulmonary leads (II, III, and aVF)
LAA (= P **M**itrale)	⌒⌒ 0.12	∨ or ⌓	**M**-shaped, widened (≥ 0.12 second) P waves in one or more of the **m**itral leads (I, II, or aVL). Deep, negative component to the P wave in lead V_1

Figure 9-2. ECG criteria for diagnosis of RAA and LAA.

Table 9-3

Findings Suggestive of RVH in Adults

1. RAA
2. RAD or indeterminate axis
3. Incomplete RBBB (or an rSr' in lead V_1)
4. Low voltage
5. Persistent precordial S waves
6. Right ventricular strain
7. Tall R wave in lead V_1

Table 9-4

Findings Suggestive of Pulmonary Disease in Adults

1. RAA
2. RAD or indeterminate axis
3. Incomplete RBBB (or an rSr' in lead V_1)
4. Low voltage
5. Persistent precordial S waves

Note that, with the exception of the last two findings in Table 9-3 (right ventricular strain, tall R wave in lead V_1), Table 9-4 is identical to Table 9-3.

QRST Changes

Table 10-1

Suggested Approach to Systematically Assessing QRST Changes

1. Ignore lead aVR
2. Scan each of the other 11 leads for **Q waves.** Note the leads in which you find them.
3. Check for **R wave progression.**
   Does transition occur in the usual place?
   Tall R wave in lead V_1?
   rSr' pattern in lead V_1?
4. Look at all leads (except aVR) for **ST segment** and **T wave** changes.

Look for **patterns of leads** in the basic lead groups *(Table 10-2).* That is, Q waves or ST-T wave changes in leads III and aVF are much more likely to be significant if they are also found in lead II.

Table 10-2

Basic Lead Groups

Inferior leads: II, III, aVF
Septal leads: V_1, V_2
Anterior leads: V_2 to V_4
Lateral leads:
   Lateral precordial leads: V_4 to V_6
   High lateral leads: I, aVL

To diagnose **right ventricular infarction,** use a **V_4R lead** and look for evidence of acute inferior infarction on the tracing.

Table 10-3

Leads That May Normally Display Moderate- to Large-Sized Q Waves*

Lead III
Lead aVF
Lead aVL
Lead V_1 (and sometimes also lead V_2)
Lead aVR†

*NOTE: Small and narrow **normal septal q waves** are often seen in one or more of the lateral leads (I, AVL, V_4, V_5, and/or V_6) in asymptomatic individuals without heart disease.

†In general we ignore lead aVR, since it rarely contributes useful information to our interpretation.

Table 10-6

Leads That May Normally Display T Wave Inversion

Lead III
Lead aVF
Lead aVL
Lead V_1 (and sometimes also lead V_2)
Lead aVR*

*In general we ignore lead aVR, since it rarely contributes useful information to our interpretation.

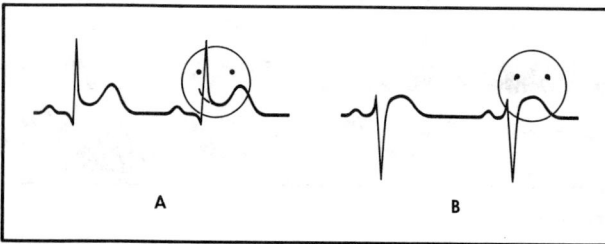

Figure 10-15. **A,** "Smiley" (upward concavity) ST segment elevation, which is usually benign, especially when it occurs in otherwise healthy, asymptomatic individuals. **B,** "Frowny" (coved) ST segment elevation, which is more often associated with acute injury from acute infarction.

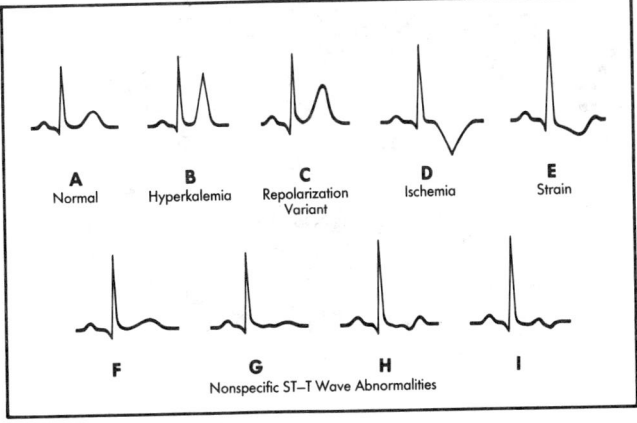

Figure 10-16. Examples of alterations in T wave morphology. **A,** Normal T wave. **B,** Tall, pointed T wave. **C,** Tall, peaked (but not pointed) T wave. **D,** Symmetrically inverted T wave. **E,** Asymmetrically inverted T wave. **F,** Slightly flattened T wave. **G,** Greater degree of T wave flattening. **H,** Biphasic T wave (initial negative component, terminal positive component). **I,** Biphasic T wave (initial positive component, terminal negative component).

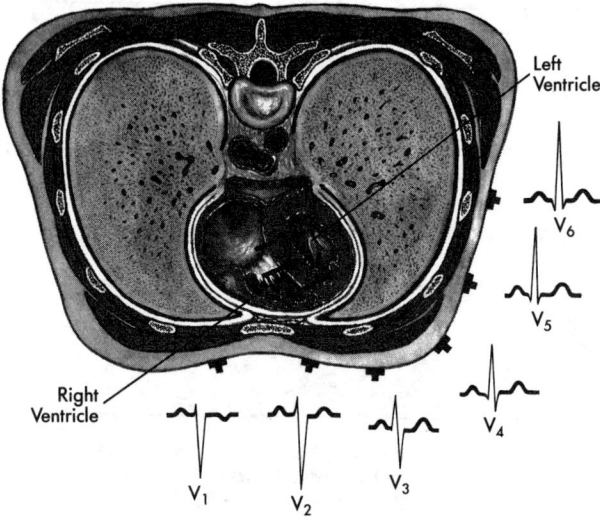

Figure 10-3. Schematic view of the heart. The arrows depict the general direction of left ventricular depolarization. The QRS complexes in the precordial leads show normal R wave progression.

Table 10-4

Common Causes of Poor R Wave Progression

LVH
RVH
Pulmonary disease (i.e., COPD, long-standing asthma)
Anterior or anteroseptal infarction
Conduction defects (i.e., LBBB, LAHB, IVCD)
Cardiomyopathy
Chest wall deformity
Normal variant
Lead misplacement

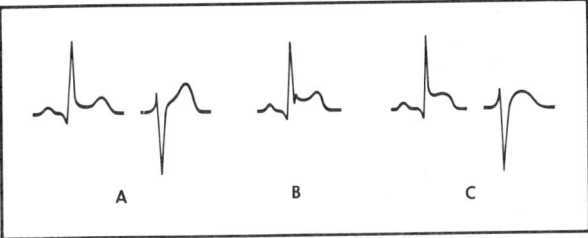

Figure 10-14. Examples of ST segment elevation. ST segment elevation with an upward concavity **(A)** tends to be benign, especially if there is J point notching **(B)**. ST segment coving **(C)** is much more likely to represent acute injury.

Infarction and Ischemia

Table 12-1

Information Sought from an ECG in Patients with Chest Pain

1. Are there acute changes?
    Is the patient likely to be infarcting? (If so, what area of the heart is likely to be involved?)
    Is there ischemia?
    Is there some other condition that might account for the ECG changes?
    Is the patient a candidate for thrombolytic therapy? (an optimal candidate?)
2. Is there evidence of prior infarction? If so, is it possible to date such changes?

Table 12-2

General Descriptors for Dating Infarction

Acute infarction: onset within hours up to a day
  ST segment elevation is hyperacute or coved, and often marked.
  Q waves are small or absent.
  T wave inversion is minimal or absent.
  Reciprocal ST segment depression is often present, and may be marked.
Old infarction: onset over a week ago
  Q waves are present and are often large.
  ST segment elevation is absent.
  T wave inversion is minimal or absent.
  There is no reciprocal ST segment depression.
Recent (i.e., **"subacute") infarction:** onset within a day or so, up to several days to a week
  Q waves are often present; they may be small or large.
  ST segment elevation is minimal or absent.
  T wave inversion is often present and may be marked.
  Reciprocal ST segment depression is minimal or absent.

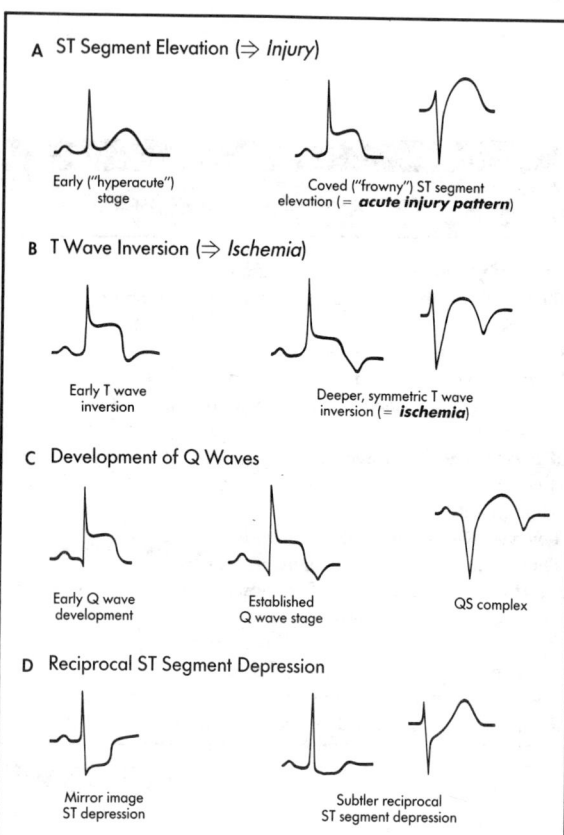

Figure 12-1. Principal ECG indicators of acute infarction.

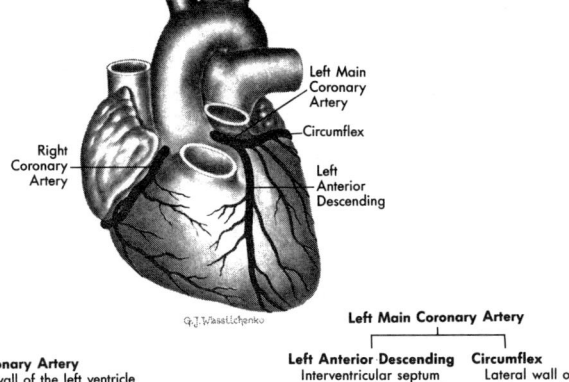

Right Coronary Artery
Inferior wall of the left ventricle
Posterior wall of the left ventricle
Right ventricle

Left Main Coronary Artery

Left Anterior Descending
Interventricular septum
Anterior wall of the left ventricle

Circumflex
Lateral wall of the left ventricle

Figure 12-3. Simplified diagram of the coronary circulation and the areas of the heart *usually* supplied by each coronary artery.

Table 12-3

Criteria for Considering Thrombolytic Therapy

Age <75 years old
History of new-onset ischemic chest pain within the "window of opportunity" (i.e., within 6 hours)
Definite ECG evidence of acute infarction
No contraindications to thrombolytic therapy

Table 12-4

Patients Likely to Benefit Most from Thrombolytic Therapy

Patients treated early
Patients with ECG evidence of large, potentially reversible infarctions:
    Anterior location
    Marked ST segment elevation
    Reciprocal ST segment depression in many leads
    Small or absent q waves

Time is the most important variable. Regarding infarction, *"time is muscle."* At present, most institutions set the upper limit of their "window of opportunity" at 6 hours. That is, symptom onset (i.e., chest pain) must have begun less than 6 hours ago for a patient to qualify as a potential candidate for thrombolytic therapy. Simply stated, *the sooner the thrombolytic therapy is started, the greater the chance that the patient will benefit.* This is especially true if thrombolytic therapy is begun within 3 hours of symptom onset.

The second major variable determining the likely benefit from thrombolytic therapy is the extent of the infarct. *The larger the infarct, the greater the potential benefit.* The ECG initially recorded at the time the patient presents can be extremely helpful in predicting the relative size of the infarct. In general, anterior infarcts are larger than inferior infarcts. The more leads that demonstrate ST segment elevation, and the greater the degree of that ST segment elevation, the larger the infarct is likely to be. This is especially true when *in addition* to ST segment elevation there is also marked reciprocal ST segment depression in multiple leads. Although Q waves do not exclude potential benefit from the thrombolytic therapy, the presence of large new Q waves makes it much less likely that myocardial damage will be reversible. Optimally, Q waves will be either absent or small at the time the patient presents.

The Five Essential Lists

We advocate recall of five essential lists in electrocardiography. We define a "list" as a series of conditions to consider in the differential diagnosis of a certain electrocardiographic finding. As soon as you recognize the finding, a "light bulb" should go off, prompting you to run through the entities in the list to see if any might be present. The purpose of making a list is simply to prevent you from overlooking a potentially important ECG diagnosis.

Table 13-2

List #1: Causes of a Regular, Wide-Complex Tachycardia

1. Ventricular tachycardia
2. VENTRICULAR TACHYCARDIA
3. **VENTRICULAR TACHYCARDIA**
4. SVT with preexisting bundle branch block
5. SVT with aberrant conduction

Assume that the cause of any regular, wide-complex tachycardia in which sinus P waves are absent (or uncertain) is VT until proven otherwise.

> *If the heart rate is under 100 beats/minute, the QT interval is probably prolonged if it is greater than HALF of the R-R interval.*

Table 13-3

List # 2: Common Causes of QT Prolongation

1. **Drugs**
    Type IA antiarrhythmic agents (i.e., quinidine, procainamide, disopyramide)
    Tricyclic antidepressants
    Phenothiazines
2. **"Lytes"**
    Hypokalemia
    Hypomagnesemia
    Hypocalcemia
3. **CNS**
    Stroke
    Intracerebral or brainstem bleeding
    Coma

NOTE: Ischemia, infarction, and/or bundle branch block may also prolong the QT interval. However, the presence of these other conditions will usually be obvious from inspection of the ECG ⇒ *If the QT interval is prolonged in the absence of QRS widening, ischemia, or infarction, think **"Drugs/Lytes/CNS"** as the cause!*

Table 13-4

List # 3: Common Causes of ST Segment Depression

1. Ischemia
2. Strain
3. Digitalis effect
4. Hypokalemia/hypomagnesemia
5. Rate-related changes
6. Any combination of the above

Table 13-5

List # 4: Common Causes of a Tall R Wave in Lead V_1

1. Wolff-Parkinson-White (WPW) syndrome
2. Right bundle branch block (RBBB)
3. Right ventricular hypertrophy (RVH)
4. Posterior MI
5. Normal variant

Table 13-6

Helpful Clues for Determining the Cause of a Tall R Wave in Lead V_1

1. **WPW:**
    QRS widening
    Short PR interval
    Delta waves (which may be positive or negative)
2. **RBBB:**
    QRS widening (≥ 0.11 second)
    rSR′ (or RBBB equivalent pattern) in lead V_1
    Wide, terminal S wave in leads I and V_6
3. **RVH:**
    Normal QRS duration
    RAA
    RAD or indeterminate axis
    Low voltage
    Persistent precordial S waves
    Right ventricular strain
4. **Posterior MI:**
    Normal QRS duration
    Evidence of inferior infarction
    Positive "mirror test"
5. **Normal variant:**
    Normal QRS duration
    Diagnosed by exclusion in the *absence* of evidence of WPW, RBBB, RVH, or posterior MI
    Often found in an otherwise healthy young adult

Table 13-7

List # 5 Causes of Anterior ST Segment Depression in the Setting of Acute Inferior Infarction

1. Reciprocal changes
2. Concomitant anterior ischemia
3. Posterior infarction
4. Any combination of the above

None of the standard precordial leads directly views the posterior wall of the left ventricle. Electrocardiographic changes that occur in the posterior wall of the left ventricle must therefore be inferred from *indirect* observation. This may be done by application of the mirror test.

Figure 13-12. Application of the **mirror test.** The test is helpful in patients with acute inferior infarction when you also suspect posterior infarction. **A,** Schematic 12-lead ECG with changes suggestive of acute inferior infarction in lead III. There is a tall R wave in lead V_1, and ST segment depression in the anterior leads (V_1, V_2, and V_3). **B,** The tracing is flipped over. Looking *through* the paper as it is held up to the light, one would now see Q waves and ST segment elevation in leads V_1, V_2, and V_3. This is a *positive mirror test,* and suggests that the anterior lead changes in **A** reflect associated acute posterior infarction.

Electrolyte Disturbances

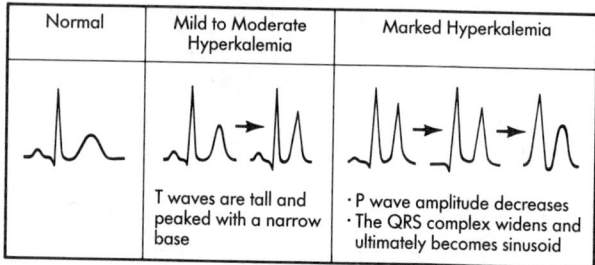

Figure 14-1. ECG manifestations of hyperkalemia.

Table 14-1

Common Clinical Settings Likely to Produce Hyperkalemia

Acute renal failure
Chronic renal failure (less common)
Acidosis
Patients taking potassium-retaining diuretics or angiotensin-converting enzyme (ACE) inhibitors
Dehydration

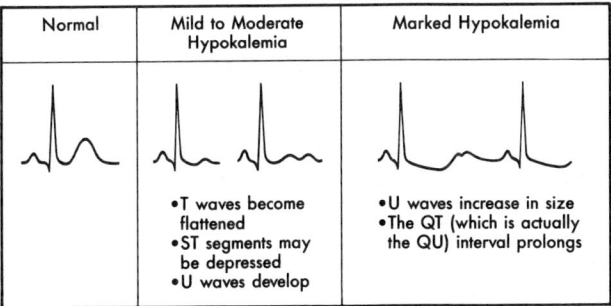

Figure 14-2. ECG manifestations of hypokalemia.

Pericarditis

The easiest way to remember the ECG manifestations of acute pericarditis is to think of them as occurring in four stages:

Stage 1: everything is UP
Stage 2: transition
Stage 3: everything is DOWN
Stage 4: normalization

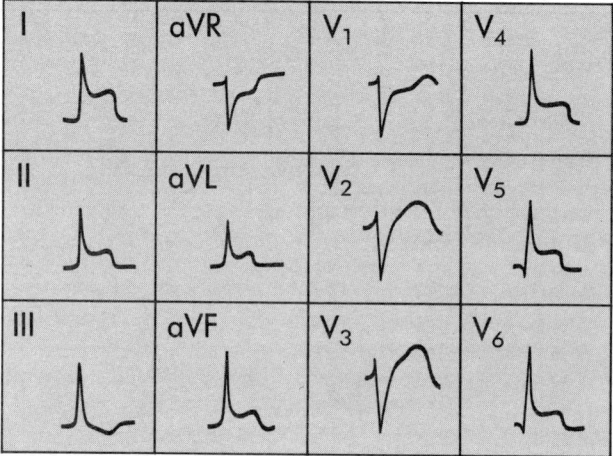

Figure 15-1. Stage 1 of acute pericarditis. There is diffuse ST segment elevation ("*everything up*" stage) in virtually all leads except aVR, V₁, and III.

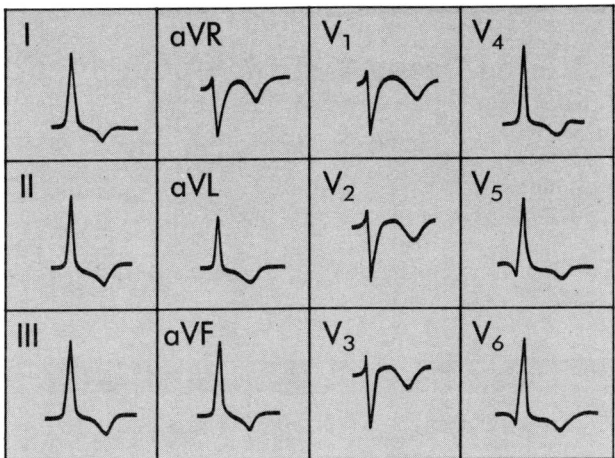

Figure 15-2. Stage 3 of acute pericarditis. Generalized ST segment elevation has been replaced by generalized T wave inversion (*"everything down"* stage).

Recognizing Lead Misplacement

Table 16-1

Findings Suggestive of Limb Lead Misplacement

A negative P wave in lead II
"Global negativity" (of the P wave, QRS complex, and T wave) in lead I
An upright QRS complex in lead aVR

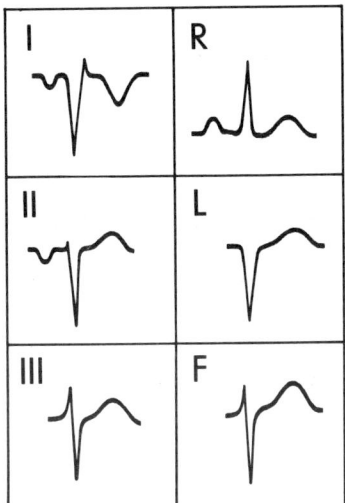

Figure 16-1. Schematic illustration of how lead misplacement in the six standard leads might look. The left and right arm electrodes have been mistakenly interchanged.

There are three clues for detecting lead misplacement in the six standard leads:

Hint to clue #1: Is the mechanism of the rhythm sinus?
Hint to clue #2: What should the QRS complex normally look like in lead I?
Hint to clue #3: What should the QRS complex normally look like in lead aVR?

When the Patient is a Child

Table 17-2

Normal Rhythm and Axis Findings in Children

Rhythm

Sinus arrhythmia is exceedingly common, especially in older children.

Sinus "tachycardia" must be redefined in children (see Table 17-1).

Axis

Pediatric norms for mean QRS axis are often much more *rightward* than for adults:

Age	Approximate normal axis deviation
Up to 30 days	Up to 180°
Up to 1 year	Up to 120°
Up to 16 years	Up to 100°

Table 17-1

Pediatric Norms for Heart Rate and Intervals

Age	Upper normal heart rate limit	Upper normal PR interval limit	Upper normal QRS duration
Newborn to 1 year	180 beats/min	≈ 0.17 second	≈ 0.08 second
1-3 years	150 beats/min	≈ 0.17 second	≈ 0.08 second
4-10 years	130 beats/min	≈ 0.17 second	≈ 0.09 second
>10 years	110 beats/min	≈ 0.20 second	≈ 0.09 second
Adults	99 beats/min	≈ 0.20-0.21 second	≈ 0.10 second

Table 17-3

Greatly Simplified Voltage Criteria for Diagnosing RVH and LVH in Children

For diagnosis of RVH

Age	Maximum allowable R wave in lead V_1	Maximum allowable S wave in lead V_6
Up to 1 month	30 mm	15 mm
1 month to 16 years	20 mm	6 mm

For diagnosis of LVH

Age	Maximum allowable S wave in lead V_1	Maximum allowable R wave in lead V_5	Maximum allowable R wave in lead V_6
Up to 12 months	20 mm	30 mm	20 mm
1-16 years	30 mm	40 mm	25 mm

When 12 Leads are Better than One

12 leads are often a lot better than one.

Evaluation of the rhythm in a single monitoring lead is often not adequate to determine the etiology of a tachycardia

Upright deflections may for all the world appear to be P waves in one lead, but in reality form part of the QRS complex.

If a portion of the QRS complex lies on the baseline, the QRS may appear deceptively narrow in that monitoring lead.

If the QRS complex is wide (so that you have a wide-complex tachycardia without definite atrial activity), *ventricular tachycardia must be assumed until proven otherwise!*

Hemodynamic status is not a helpful clue to the etiology of a tachycardia.

Assessment of QRS morphology may be an invaluable clue!

Assessment of QRS axis sometimes provides additional information.

Table 19-1

Reasons Why 12 Leads are Better than One

Optimizes evaluation of atrial activity

Provides a look at the *KEY LEADS:*
  Lead II
  Lead V_1
  Any of the other 10 leads on the ECG that show P waves
CLINICAL APPLICATION:
  For regular rhythms with a narrow QRS—may allow differentiation between sinus tachycardia, PSVT, and atrial flutter
  For regular rhythms with a wide QRS—may allow differentiation between SVT and ventricular tachycardia
  For irregular rhythms—may allow differentiation between atrial fibrillation, multifocal atrial tachycardia (MAT), and sinus rhythm with multiple PACs

Optimizes assessment of QRS morphology

Provides a look at the *KEY LEADS*:*
  Lead V_1 (or MCL_1) and lead V_6 (or MCL_6)
CLINICAL APPLICATION:
  Differentiation of PVCs from aberrantly conducted beats
  Differentiation of ventricular tachycardia from SVT

*Lead II is *not* a useful lead for evaluating QRS morphology!

Table 19-1

Reasons Why 12 Leads are Better than One—cont'd

Allows determination of QRS axis

Provides a look at the *KEY LEADS* for axis determination (leads I, II, and aVF)

CLINICAL APPLICATION:
  The finding of either marked RAD or marked LAD strongly suggests ventricular tachycardia.

Allows verification of changes seen in one lead

CHANGES SEEN/CLINICAL APPLICATION:
  ST segment elevation ⇒ Suspect development of acute injury/infarction or coronary spasm
  ST segment depression ⇒ Suspect development of ischemia (silent ischemia?) or infarction
  A shift in axis ⇒ Suspect development of LAHB (when net QRS deflection in lead II suddenly becomes predominantly negative)
  A change in QRS morphology ⇒ Suspect development of bundle branch block or a change in the site of impulse formation

	Suggestive of a SUPRAVENTRICULAR Etiology/Aberration	Of NO HELP in Differentiation	Suggestive of a VENTRICULAR Etiology
Right-sided monitoring leads (such as V$_1$ or MCL$_1$)	Taller <u>RIGHT</u> rabbit ear A B	Taller <u>RIGHT</u> rabbit ear C D E	Taller <u>LEFT</u> rabbit ear F G H
Left-sided monitoring leads (such as I, V$_5$, V$_6$ or MCL$_6$)	I J	K	L M

Figure 19B-4. Differentiation of wide beats **when the QRS complex is upright in V$_1$.**

	Suggestive of a SUPRAVENTRICULAR Etiology/Aberration	Of NO HELP in Differentiation	Suggestive of a VENTRICULAR Etiology
Right-sided monitoring leads (such as V$_1$ or MCL$_1$)	N O		P Q
Left-sided monitoring leads (such as I, V$_5$, V$_6$ or MCL$_6$)	R S		T U V

Figure 19B-5. Differentiation of wide beats **when the QRS complex is negative in V$_1$.**